Business and Pump

DEDICATED

to all those who use it and make it their own.

CONTENT

What do you prefer?
Preventive training and activity, or
the consequences of inactivity?

"Mind and body go together" – this saying is often used but is rarely effectively or efficiently applied.

Especially for today's productive appliers, the focus in everyday life is mainly on business.

Should I take the stairs today, rather than the lift? Go for a jog after work? Good ideas – but most people find that motivation flags after just a short while.

Why is that? What's missing is the result, the concrete productivity, the variety and the visible success.

But this can be changed!

This muscle guide is based on strategies and foundations derived from practice that will help you to develop, promote and support your body as well as your business and your income.

It is not a collection of literature; it is based on experience, is functional and will give more power to your life.

To whom is it addressed? To all those who apply.

The best tip, besides this book? Work with an experienced, successful coach!

And now: Let's go!

THE FOUNDATION

The foundation is the base of every structure. It is what supports all the other elements, from the steel beams to the roof, that will eventually form the finished building. The most amazing structures in the world can be built on the foundation – think of the Burj Khalifa in Dubai, in the United Arab Emirates. The foundation is the base and the precondition for sustainable, long-lasting success.

Let us now examine the two most important construction materials that make up the foundation, in this case our mindset (attitude).

ATTITUDE

Your attitude is the absolutely basic precondition to act in a future-oriented manner.
Since you are an applier, I assume that you know what I'm talking about. A clear focus, positivity and hunger are essential preconditions to adapt your body to your mental sharpness.

How can attitude be changed?

It is important to realise that our attitude is always based on a decision. Sometimes it's conscious, sometimes unconscious. We can always decide what our attitude is. We do this by first becoming aware of what or who is influencing us and of what we can change so that this input supports us in our project. Once we become aware of this fact, it becomes obvious that we can adjust our attitude, and allow ourselves to be influenced, as we desire.

PS: You've already been doing this. Test this statement: what is your attitude after listing to a specific tune that is upbeat? Usually the answer is: you also feel upbeat.

It is therefore absolutely essential to adjust your own attitude positively to your long-term success and your goals.

Power Tip

Surround yourself with people who have goals, avoid useless information and actively soak up informative, productive knowledge.

What are your goals?

YOUR GOALS

You should set the bar high with regard to bodybuilding, because here as in other things, it's important to think big!

Even if your main focus is on your business projects, it is important to expand the previous expectations for your goal. Think in terms of top-flight bodybuilding, follow the best athletes on social media, and new paths and possibilities will present themselves to you.

One good reference point is the most prestigious event in body-building, Mister Olympia, and the people who participate in it, many of whom have a social media presence. Through conscious, and also unconscious, information exchange you can obtain many tips and better visualise your own goals. Learn from the best!

For your information: the "Mr. O" event takes place annually in the USA.

It is important that you simultaneously specify and visualise your goals. Concretely, you can set a target weight that you wish to achieve by a certain point in time. But note: building muscle and fitness are not directly correlated.

Depending on your current body shape, you may for example have to gain a significant amount of weight, rather than lose it, in the medium term. If you judge your body fat percentage to be low, set a much higher weight as your goal.

If you need advice in this regard, ideally you should ask a coach or more advanced athletes in the gym, and pay special attention to the following tips regarding the right nutrition.

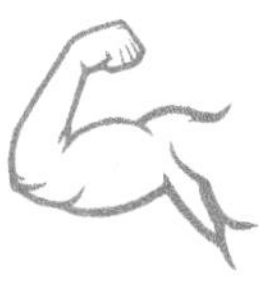

Power Tip

Every morning, make an overview of your goals and projects. Do this not just for your business activities but for all areas of your life, including your health and your body. Add this to your morning routine and you will be amazed at how little priority you assigned to your body before – and how much you do now!

Ask yourself:
What am I currently perceiving?
Is this input useful for my goals?

THE THREE STEEL PILLARS
THE TRIANGLE OF HEALTHY SPORTS

THE TRAINING

How should you design your customised workout programme?

First analyse how much time you can – and more importantly, want to – invest in your body every week.

You should choose a value that you can actually achieve every week, including in weeks and on individual days on which you dedicate a lot of time to your business activities.

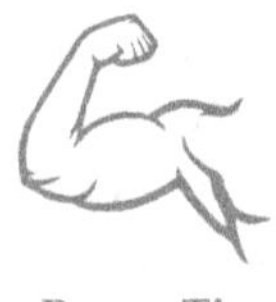

Power Tip

Give your body four hours a week and it will thank you.

This represents less than 2.4 per cent of your week. It's a high-yield investment.

How should you concretely shape your workout schedule?

Given the suggestion above, your training could consist of three weight training units of around one hour each. Use the fourth unit for a cardio session or split it into active stretching and the corresponding cardio unit.

What exercises should you do?

In the scheme above, you would train following the upper body/ lower body principle. This means that you train the muscles in your upper body in the first unit of the week and then focus on your lower body in the following unit. In the third and last unit of the week, you then do upper body training again. The following week, you start with a lower body workout in the first unit, so that the training days take place in alternation.

You should focus on the basic moves of weight training, which are as follows:

Bench press
Deadlift
Squats
Overhead press
Pull-ups
Fly (Lateral lift)
Dips (strategically, these are not included in the following training plan)

It is essential that you first learn to do these exercises with a clean technique before increasing the weights for the individual exercises. Get advice from experienced, more advanced athletes in the gym, or ideally from a trainer. You can also find suitable training videos online. The (basic) exercises above have the advantage that they primarily train one muscle while also using other muscle groups as support and stabilisation when done correctly. As a result, these are also trained.

You've certainly already seen that in gyms people use barbells, dumbbells and machines. All instruments are useful and have their individual benefits. Working with free weights usually requires stabilisation and coordination effort, while machine training defines the scope of movement and better isolates and trains the respective muscles.

Combine free weights and machine training.

In this way you will make the best of both worlds.

It is important that you do not just do the exercise across the whole range of movement but rather focus on using the targeted muscles. One frequently sees people using mostly their arms for the overhead press when in fact these are secondary to the actual target muscle group, the shoulders.

The following table shows which are the working muscles for each exercise:

Exercise	Primary muscles	Secondary muscles
Bench press	Chest muscles	Triceps, front shoulder
Deadlift, stretched	Biceps femoris muscle	Lower back, forearms
Squats	Leg muscles	Buttocks
Overhead press	Shoulder muscles	Upper chest, triceps
Pull-ups	Back muscles	Biceps, forearms
Dips	Depending on execution: - chest muscles - triceps	Front shoulder

Inclined bench press	Chest muscles	Triceps, front shoulder
Rowing	Back muscles	Biceps, forearms
Fly (Lateral lift)	Side shoulder muscles	
Face pulls	Back shoulder muscles	

The following workout plan is an example and can be adapted to your preferences, because fun is an essential part of training if you want long-term success in reaching your goals. If you have never done bodybuilding exercises before, you could start exclusively on machines to develop your muscle feel (your "muscle-mind connection"). There are also additional options to design your training. Look into the push-pull training plan, for instance.

Do you have individual preferences? Ideally, you should try to ask an experienced trainer, who can help you with both the theory and the practice.

EXAMPLE WORKOUT PLAN 1

Warm-up:
→ Move body (e.g. 5-10 minutes crosstrainer)
→ Mobilise body (if required)
→ Increase the training weights up to the final working weight (around two sets)

1st set: 6-15 reps with 40% - 50% of the working weight
2nd set: 6-15 reps with 60% - 70% of the working weight

UPPER BODY

Exercise	Equipment	Sets x reps
Chest press	Machine	3 x 12
Side rowing	Machine	3 x 8
Overhead press	Dumbbells	3 x 8
Pull-ups/lat pull	Free/machine	3 x 8
Fly (Lateral lift)	Dumbbells	2 x 12
10 min. cool-down cardio		
Bonus tip: Frequently expand the plan by adding a column in your notes (the weight you're currently using).		

LOWER BODY

Exercise	Equipment	Sets x reps
Squats/leg press	Barbell/machine	3 x 10
Stretched deadlift	Barbell/dumbbells	3 x 8
Leg extension	Machine	3 x 8
Belly crunches	Free/machine	2 x 12
10 min. cool-down cardio		
Bonus tip: Frequently expand the plan by adding a column in your notes (the weight you're currently using).		

Exercise	Equipment	Duration
Cycling	-	30 min.

My advice is to start with one set less at first but to slightly increase the number of reps, before gradually shifting to the numbers in the plan. Use a training weight with which you can do almost or exactly as many reps, with the proper technique, as prescribed in the plan and try to increase in every workout unit: whether increasing the training weight by the smallest denominator, or a few reps more with the current weight, until you have reached the desired number of reps. The exercises can be replaced without problems, especially in the medium term.

The training days could be as follows: Monday (upper body), Wednesday (lower body), Friday (upper body), Sunday (cardio). In the following week, start with the lower body workout system.

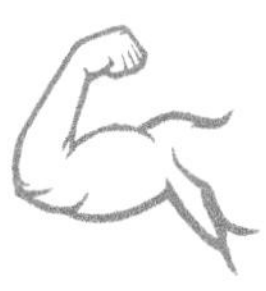

Power Tip

Keep a training diary. Simply copy the plan above into a document in which you can adjust the training values (e.g. Microsoft Excel/Word).

At each workout, open a note on your smartphone and enter your current values. After the workout, transfer them to the document. There are also apps that help you do this. This ensures that you maintain an overview and full control of your progress.

What should I do if I would like to work out a bit more or more often?

My advice is to not significantly exceed the training scope above. During the workout unit you use your muscles and set a +certain impulse so that they can regenerate a little more strongly in the regeneration phase and so are ready more quickly and can perform better. When you increase the number of sets or reps, you often reach a phase of "overtraining", with reduced regeneration capacity.
But what you want is the best and most efficient results!
Also note that as you progress, your training volume (training volume = sets x reps x weight) increases.

Of course there are also other methods to design your workout. For instance, the individual muscle groups can be trained just once or several times during the week.
If you want to invest in your body every day, I advise you to increase the number of cardio or active stretching units. Alternatively, ask an experienced trainer for a plan that is adjusted to more units per week, with the training volume correspondingly spread out.

If the plan above already gives you the feeling that your regeneration is insufficient, only use machines for the exercises and test if your regeneration improves. If you can, ask an experienced, successful trainer on site for advice.

What should I do if I don't want to work out more than twice per week?

My personal advice is to go for a "full body workout" in which you train all your muscles in the first training unit of the week and

repeat this in the second, ideally with different exercises. A cardio unit should be added on to every workout unit.
Alternatively, do your cardio training as a separate, third unit. Naturally this can also take place outside the gym.

The following plan is an example for a "full body workout":

EXAMPLE WORKOUT PLAN 2

Warm-up:
→ Move body (e.g. 5-10 minutes cross-trainer)
→ Mobilise body (if required)
→ Increase the training weights up to the final working weight (around two sets)
1st set: 6-15 reps with 40% - 50% of the working weight
2nd set: 6-15 reps with 60% - 70% of the working weight

FULL BODY 1.1

Exercise	Equipment	Sets x reps
Squats/leg press	Barbell/machine	3 x 12
Overhead press	Dumbbells	3 x 10
Pull-ups/lat pulls	Free/machine	3 x 10
Fly (Lateral lift)	Dumbbells	2 x 12
10 min. cool-down cardio		

Bonus tip: Frequently expand the plan by adding a column in your notes (the weight you're currently using).

Exercise	Equipment	Sets x reps
Bench press	Barbell	3 x 10
Stretched deadlift	Barbell/dumbbells	3 x 12
Dips	Free/machine	3 x 10
Belly crunches	Free/machine	2 x 12
10 min. cool-down cardio		
Bonus tip: Frequently expand the plan by adding a column in your notes (the weight you're currently using).		

CARDIO

Exercise	Equipment	Duration
Cycling	-	30 min.

Why is training the back and the back shoulders so important?

Since your main focus is your business, I assume that you spend a lot of your day sitting. To train an upright, straight and stable body posture it is important to actively use the respective muscles. The plans above take this into account. If you want to further focus on your back shoulders, face pulls or reverse butterfly exercises are recommended.

What should my stretching programme look like concretely?

First, it is important to emphasise that stretching and mobilising, in contrast to muscle building training, serves not to tense the muscles but to relax them.

I'm sure you already know some basic stretching moves. Those are the most effective anyway. A brief online search will throw up some more helpful tips.
With stretching as with working out, you should take care to build up gradually, for instance by increasing the range of the movement. However, progress here is not as relevant is progress in active muscle training.

The duration of mobilisation can be 15 to 30 minutes based on your preference. This includes stretching the upper and lower body. Assigning much longer to this is usually not necessary.

Keep it simple! Use one of the plans provided here and ask advanced athletes or a trainer for advice regarding how to execute the exercises and about your progress.

Make sure that you do your training in that hour of the day that is best suited to you. After the workout, it's back to your other priorities.

Power Tip

Move a lot!

NUTRITION

You should adjust your nutrition to your new, or improved, lifestyle.

But note that you should avoid any radical, precisely scheduled nutrition plan if you're not actually actively doing bodybuilding.

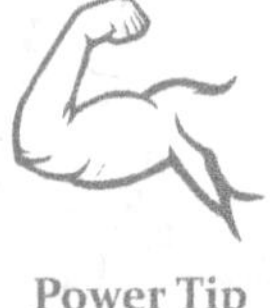

Avoid extreme eating habits. The foundations and solid basics are what your advantages should be variably and flexibly adjusted to.

What food groups are there, and which ones are relevant?

Carbohydrates, around 4 kcal/1 g
Proteins, around 4 kcal/1 g
Fats, around 9 kcal/1 g
Vitamins
Minerals
Water

Carbohydrates, proteins and fats are macronutrients and can provide you with significant amounts of energy. Vitamins and minerals are called micronutrients. It is important to remember that all the food groups cited above are important for your health and for your body's performance, often in combination.

Whether you gain or lose weight depends mainly on whether you take up more calories over a certain period of time than you expend (weight gain) or fewer calories than you expend (weight loss).

It is therefore also possible to lose weight while exclusively eating very fatty foods, provided that your intake is below your general calorie requirements. Of course doing so is not helpful to a healthily functioning body in the long run. However, healthy fats in particular are also essential nutrients that you should not avoid in your food.

What about proteins?

As you certainly know, proteins are an important component of muscle growth.
You have probably already bought a so-called protein bar in the supermarket or drugstore, assuming that you are doing something good for your body.

And there certainly are protein bars with good nutritional values. However, you should make sure that they have a low sugar content and that the proteins are from a suitable source that the body can easily absorb. The following are generally recommended, regardless of whether they're in a protein bar or in a similar product: whey protein concentrates and whey product isolates (animal origin), and proteins from rice or peas (vegetable origin). But since the available protein bars rarely have a good price-quality ratio, I rather recommend using a protein powder made from the sources above to mix in water or milk.

Should I consume nutritional supplements, and if yes, which ones?

Generally speaking, nutritional supplements are an addition to your food, as their name already suggests. Their role is to guarantee in a practical way that your body gets the appropriate nutrients over the course of the day.

However, these nutrients can also be taken up without supplements, as part of your diet. Taking supplements is therefore purely optional and depends on your specific diet.

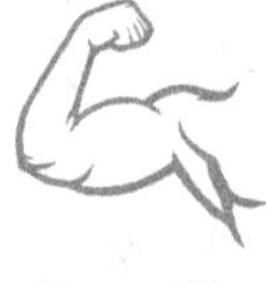

Power Tip

Get your hands on a protein powder of vegetable or animal origin. On workout days, prepare yourself a mixed shake for optimum nutrient supply after training, and repeat this on non-workout days at a time of your choosing.

Optionally, you can supplement your diet with a multi-vitamin preparation and also an omega-3 supplement. The latter is available both as fish oil and as algae oil (vegan alternative), usually in the form of capsules. Go for the products of accredited manufacturers if you can, to be sure that they follow high standards in production.

It is generally recommended to enrich these with a bit of salt at the corresponding meals.

Try to ensure that every one of your meals contains a bit of protein.

What should I eat after the workout?

After the workout, it is especially important to supply the body with new energy and nutrients. The so-called glycogen stores also need to be replenished. Beside the classic protein shake, a carbohydrate meal is therefore recommended.

What foodstuffs should form the basis of my diet?

Recommended foodstuffs are predominantly "living" ones – mostly unprocessed foods that we already know are basic foodstuffs.

The following table provides recommendations for choosing your macronutrients with the respective primary foodstuffs that contain them:

Carbohydrates	Proteins	Fats
Rice	Seeds (various)	Nuts
Potatoes	Beans	Cheese
(Whole grain) pasta	Broccoli	Peanut butter
Oats	Peas	Olives
Whole grain bread	Eggs (watch the fats)	Avocado
Whole grain toast	Nuts (watch the fats)	Linseed oil
Rice puffs	Cheese (watch the fats)	
Honey	Peanut butter (watch the fats)	
Bananas	Fish e.g. salmon	
	Meat e.g. chicken, turkey, beef	

You should also supplement your diet with copious amounts of fruits and vegetables. Every now and then, you can also treat yourself to food that is considered "unhealthy". This will not harm your body composition if you maintain the workout regimen.

An important point: develop the habit of having healthy food as your basic diet. Put together meals in which you combine different nutrients.

How much fluid should I drink?

If possible, drink around one litre (= 33.81 us fl oz) per 20 kilos (= 44,09 lb) of body weight. If you weigh 80 kilos (= 176,37 lb) and you work out, that's four litres. But if the actual value is a little under the recommendation, that's not a problem. Here as in other things, you should listen to your body.

REGENERATION

Regeneration is also a decisive factor with regard to building up your muscles and your general performance.

Frequently excessively training the same muscles is a common error when starting bodybuilding. However, this depends greatly on the individual. You should therefore test for yourself after a few weeks if the workout plans presented above are really optimised for you or if you should adjust the volume downwards or even upwards.

As a general rule, you should bear in mind that your muscles build up in those phases in which you are not training and that they can adjust to the load. In the best case, they even regenerate a bit more strongly than was the case before training. This effect, which was already mentioned above, is known as super-compensation.

Note: bodybuilding to achieve very large muscles does not occur in a few weeks, but rather over months or even years. But workout

beginners will very quickly see improvements.
Make use of this advantage!

How much sleep should I get for optimal regeneration?

Depending on what's possible for you, sleeping for seven to nine hours is recommended.

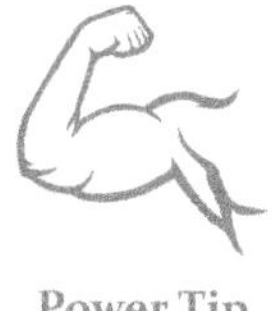

The golden mean is probably the safest bet. Eight hours are ideal; but it depends both on your personal preference and on your possibilities.

Is the additional cardio training nevertheless recommended for my regeneration?

Definitely. As long as you don't squeeze in excessive amounts of cardio and endurance training in addition to the workout plans above, additional cardio training can even improve your regeneration.
Furthermore, you will be actively doing something for your circulation, your entire skeleton and muscles, your stamina, and will be giving your body many other positive benefits.
If you can, get advice from an experienced trainer who believes in and executes both forms, weight training and endurance sport.

Are there any more tips for a refreshing sleep?

Yes there are; check out the following Power Tip!

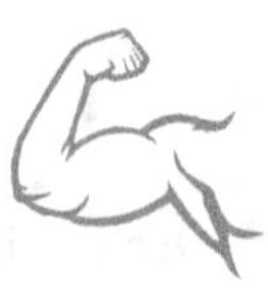

Avoid bright screens around one hour before you go to bed. Most smartphones have a feature that reduces the bright blue light.

Power Tip

Supply your body with nutrients, follow the tips in 1.1 and visualise your goals.

THE TWO IRRELEVANT STEEL PILLARS

Previously we looked at how you can discover your customised workout plan and where you can get additional information. We focused on the foundations and the most important factors for power nutrition and also just analysed regeneration and its essential properties.

For the sake of completeness, I will now also mention two other pillars that are often referred to in high-performance sport. However, they should be of little significance to you.

The fourth pillar is your genes. In professional bodybuilding, this is often a decisive factor. Being a presentation sport, in bodybuilding athletes are often compared to a specific optimal image. This often includes a particularly thin waist and broad shoulders.
But since you cannot directly influence these factors, and since your primary focus is on your business anyway, this aspect is not relevant to you. Furthermore, you are an individual, and you are improving your body for your own sake.

The fifth and final pillar is performance-enhancing support, in which certain substances, according to the myth, are used not as intended but in this case to grow more muscle.

Since using these can come with a large number of negative health effects, consuming them at the time you start training is not very useful, and your focus is not on top-flight bodybuilding anyway, I strongly advise against using such substances.

You should always discuss individual points regarding your health with your doctor, and also with your coach if it is warranted.

APPLICATION

CREATING TIME, INTEGRATING INTO DAILY ROUTINE

Now that you have acquired some theoretical knowledge about the proper power mindset and about bodybuilding, we will look more closely at the practical application.

Once you have concretised and visualised your goals, you will realise that you do not need to manage the time you invest in sports. Rather, you can create it.

How come?

Comparably to your business activities, you now assign a new, higher priority to your health and your body.

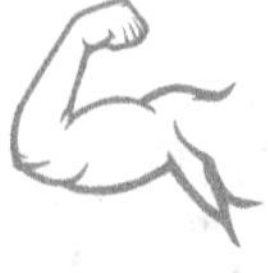

Make use of the momentum of your day and have your workout. After one hour, leave the gym, ideally having set new records, and continue your day's schedule.

Power Tip — Remember: you're working for yourself.

Can I replace the cardio units at the gym with cycling in nature?

Of course! In fact, that is the superior option. The fresh air and the natural surroundings will definitely do your body good. Fast walking and other indoor and outdoor activities in or outside the gym are also highly recommended. Listen to your body and act according to your individual preferences.

THE PLAN

Now that you have the firm conviction that you can acquire further information as well as practical tips for your successful workout, you are probably wondering about what concrete actions to take next.

These are listed below:

1. Read this work again. Highlight the important tips.

2. Add an overview of your projects to your morning routine. Include in it your new health package with its three most important pillars.

3. Sign up at a gym today. Yes, today! If you are already signed up, ask yourself the following questions: What is the price-quality ratio? Is the gym conveniently located near me?

4. Select your workout plan based on your individual preferences. If you can, get in touch with a coach. The help of a coach is especially valuable in the beginning. Ideally he should be successful in the field and should already have worked with non-supporting athletes.

5. Do you already follow successful athletes on their social media channels?

6. Apply! You can always make adjustments at a later time.

7. Once you achieve some success: help those around you and pass on your practical and theoretical knowledge.

8. I would be very happy to receive feedback on your success.
Do you have more workout plans to share with the community?
Let us know about them! Post them in the comments
Do you have more practical Power Tips?

I sincerely hope that you do not just apply the foundations and tips for healthy bodybuilding but also develop a real interest in the topic of movement and (weight) training. Use the tips and share your own experience.

Start today!

NOTES

LEGAL NOTICE

The contents of this work were put together with great care and were also inspected by experienced athletes. Nonetheless, there are no guarantees for it being complete, correct or up to date.

The contents are based mainly on the author's personal experiences and views.

Individual issues and preferences should always be discussed and with a trainer or a (specialised) doctor and applied accordingly.

The application of tips and workout plans is at the reader's own risk.

IMPRINT

© 2020 Benedikt Hoff

1ˢᵗ edition

Publisher: Benedikt Hoff, Beekerstraße 4, DE- 47638 Straelen
Cover design, layout: Aleksandra Lunk

The present work, including its components, is protected by copyright. Any exploitation without the publisher's consent is forbidden. This applies especially to electronic or other duplication, translation, distribution or making the work publicly accessible.

ABOUT THE AUTHOR

At just 21, Benedikt Hoff has been bodybuilding for more than six years. In this time he has collected a body of knowledge of which he is sure that it is largely relevant to many other people.

In particular, the foundations of a practical, healthy diet should form the basis of (almost) every person's eating habits. One important insight: unhealthy foods do not need to be completely eliminated from the diet and can even provide the body with energy.

No carbohydrates after 18:00? The author believes that it is possible to lose weight even if one only eats carbohydrates after 18:00.

He is particularly practice-focused and advises his readers to continue to develop themselves and make their own individual experiences.